introducing ophthalmology

A PRIMER FOR OFFICE STAFF

Second Edition

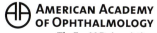

AMERICAN ACADEMY OF OPHTHALMOLOGY
The Eye M.D. Association

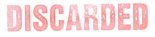

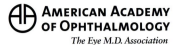
AMERICAN ACADEMY
OF OPHTHALMOLOGY
The Eye M.D. Association

655 Beach Street
P.O. Box 7424
San Francisco, CA 94120-7424

11-12

introducing ophthalmology

11-12 DO

ALLIED HEALTH EDUCATION COMMITTEE
Tyree Carr, MD, Chair
Peter C. Donshik, MD
Andrew G. Lee, MD
Elbert Magoon, MD
Emanuel Newmark, MD
Ralph S. Sando, MD
Donna Applegate, COT, Consultant
Lindreth DuBois, MEd, MMSc, COMT, Consultant
Kate Goldblum, RN, Consultant

ACADEMY STAFF
Richard A. Zorab, Vice President,
    Ophthalmic Knowledge
Hal Straus, Director of Publications
William M. Hering, PhD, Director of Programs
Carol L. Dondrea, Program Manager,
    Allied Health Education
Ruth Modric, Production Manager
Socorro Soberano, Designer

Printed in China
06 05   5 4 3

contents

Chinese spectacles with tangerine skin case, ca 1780

(Courtesy Museum of Vision, Foundation of the American Academy of Ophthalmology)

preface

This second edition of *Introducing Ophthalmology: A Primer for Office Staff* has been updated, with a new look and color illustrations. In addition, a glossary has been added to help readers quickly find the meanings of new terms. Reviewed and revised by the Allied Health Education Committee of the American Academy of Ophthalmology, this edition, like the first, serves as a basic introduction to the field of ophthalmology for clinical and nonclinical staff.

PREFACE TO THE FIRST EDITION

Everyone who works in an ophthalmology office contributes to the care of the ophthalmologist's patients. Because they help the ophthalmologist directly with patients, medical assistants and other clinical staff need a basic understanding of the specialty of ophthalmology, the workings of the eye, and common eye diseases. Because they contribute in an equally important, though indirect, way to patient care, nonclinical workers such as secretaries, billing clerks, and transcriptionists also benefit from understanding basic concepts in ophthalmology.

This booklet, developed by the Allied Health Education Committee of the American Academy of Ophthalmology, is intended to introduce new workers, both clinical and nonclinical, to some basic concepts about eyes, eye health, and the medical specialty of ophthalmology. *Introducing Ophthalmology* can help new employees feel comfortable with a new vocabulary of medical terms and can give beginning medical transcriptionists, secretaries, and clerks an insight into the new eye health concepts they encounter. Besides introducing new receptionists to the types of patient problems and medical activities that occur in an ophthalmology office, this brief book can help them communicate more effectively with patients and experienced staff alike. And it can help familiarize beginning medical assistants with the complexities of ophthalmologic conditions, tests, and procedures.

Office staff who have been on the job for a while will find much of the information in *Introducing Ophthalmology* familiar. Nevertheless, ophthalmology office workers, both experienced and inexperienced, may find the simple explanations in this booklet useful in answering patients' questions. Also helpful for office staff and patients alike are the nine Eye Myths and Facts boxes that are found throughout the booklet. These informative boxes illustrate a variety of common misconceptions about the eye and eye care and can help dispel some of the many current myths about eye health.

For readers interested in more technical information about ophthalmology and ophthalmic medical assisting, *Introducing Ophthalmology* concludes with a list of suggested resources available from the American Academy of Ophthalmology, including educational publications and videotapes. Also listed are several valuable reference books from other sources.

For those who decide to make ophthalmic medical assisting their career, two organizations are of particular importance: the Joint Commission on Allied Health Personnel in Ophthalmology (JCAHPO), the certifying body for ophthalmic medical assistants, and the Association of Technical Personnel in Ophthalmology (ATPO), the profession's national association. Contact information for both groups can be found in the Suggested Resources section.

1 introduction to

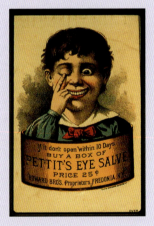

Pettit's Eye Salve, ca 1900
Trade card (front)

*(Courtesy Museum of Vision,
Foundation of the American Academy
of Ophthalmology)*

ophthalmology

WHAT IS OPHTHALMOLOGY?

The word **ophthalmology** (pronounced ahf-thahl-MOL-uh-jee) comes from the Greek word *ophthalmos,* meaning "eyeball" or "eye." Ophthalmology is the branch of medicine dealing with the eyes. Note that the word is spelled with 2 *h*'s and 2 *l*'s (Figure 1.1). Before reading any further, look away from this booklet and try spelling the word on a piece of paper. Then look back. Did you get it right?

WHAT IS AN OPHTHALMOLOGIST?

An **ophthalmologist** is a medical doctor (MD) or an osteopathic physician (DO), specially trained in the medical and surgical care and treatment of the eyes. Becoming an ophthalmologist can take 12 or more years of advanced education and training. Ophthalmologists must complete 4 years of college, 4 years of medical school, and 1 year of **internship** (hospital training). After that, the doctor undergoes 3 to 5 years of hospital **residency** to train in the medical specialty of ophthalmology.

An ophthalmologist may practice as a **comprehensive**, or **general, ophthalmologist**, a doctor who treats a wide range of eye problems and conditions. For example, patients might visit a comprehensive ophthalmologist for a routine medical eye examination, which would include having their vision checked and perhaps receiving a prescription

Figure 1.1
The word *ophthalmology* has 2 *h*'s and 2 *l*'s.

1

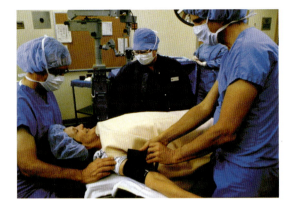

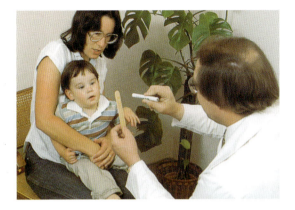

Figure 1.2 (left)
A comprehensive ophthalmologist provides a wide variety of medical eye care services, such as performing surgery on the eye and surrounding structures.

Figure 1.3 (right)
Subspecialist ophthalmologists specialize in certain areas of eye care, such as children's eye problems.

for eyeglasses or contact lenses. Patients also would visit a comprehensive ophthalmologist to have their eyes examined for a particular disease or injury and receive medication or surgical treatment (Figure 1.2).

Some ophthalmologists obtain **fellowship** training after residency to learn more about one or two specific aspects or elements of the eye. After this fellowship training, they practice as **subspecialists**, doctors who concentrate on treating eye problems primarily in those few specific areas. For example, a subspecialist may concentrate only on medical and surgical problems of the outer parts of the eye or on children's eye problems or on eye problems related to just one disease, such as glaucoma (Figure 1.3).

It may seem surprising that a doctor would require so much training to treat such a small body part. But when we consider how important vision is to us all, and how complex and delicate the eye is, it isn't so surprising after all.

WHAT OTHER PROFESSIONALS CARE FOR THE EYES?

People commonly confuse ophthalmologists with optometrists and opticians, but there are important differences among them. The main difference is that, unlike ophthalmologists, neither optometrists nor opticians are required to attend or graduate from medical school. Because they do not have a medical training or background, optometrists and opticians provide only limited forms of eye care.

Optometrists (Doctors of Optometry, or ODs) attend 4 years of college and 4 years of optometry school, where they are trained to examine the eyes to determine the presence of a limited number and type of vision problems and certain problems related to eye movement. Optometrists primarily prescribe eyeglasses and contact lenses. Some states in the United States permit optometrists to diagnose (determine the presence and nature of) certain eye diseases and treat them with mostly topical medications (eyedrops or ointment), within limitations. No state permits optometrists to perform conventional surgery.

Opticians are individuals who are trained to design, verify, and fit eyeglass lenses and frames, contact lenses, and other devices to correct eyesight. They use prescriptions supplied by ophthalmologists or optometrists, but they do not test vision or write prescriptions for visual correction. Opticians are not permitted to diagnose or treat eye diseases.

EYE MYTHS AND FACTS

Reading in poor light will hurt the eyes.
Before the invention of the electric light, most nighttime reading and other work was done by dim candlelight or gaslight. Reading in dim light today won't harm our eyes any more than it did our ancestors' eyes— or any more than taking a photograph in dim light will damage a camera.

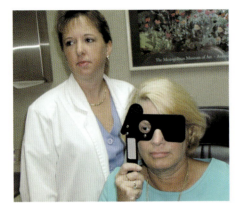

In contrast to optometrists and opticians, ophthalmologists are *medical* doctors who can examine the eyes in relation to the general health and condition of the whole body. The ophthalmologist is the only one of these three professionals who is qualified as a physician to diagnose all eye diseases and to prescribe or perform medical and surgical treatment of the eye.

Besides the ophthalmologist, many other types of workers may be found in an ophthalmology office. Some are *clinical* staff, meaning they perform technical medical duties directly associated with the care of patients. Others hold equally important but nontechnical positions. Together, these professionals form an important part of the eye care team.

Nonclinical staff may include receptionists, billing clerks, secretaries, office managers, and other workers who contribute to the smooth business operation of a medical office. In many offices or clinics, nonclinical workers speak directly with patients to make appointments, obtain insurance information, and the like. But even those workers who do not communicate with patients play an important part in overall patient care and satisfaction with treatment.

Clinical workers, sometimes referred to as **allied health personnel**, may include ophthalmic medical assistants, technicians, and technologists; ophthalmic registered nurses; orthoptists; and ophthalmic photographers. An **ophthalmic medical assistant** performs a variety of tests on patients and generally helps the doctor with the patient's medical examination and care in the office (Figure 1.4). Highly trained or experienced assistants, sometimes called *technicians* or *technologists,* may help with more complicated or technical medical tests and minor office surgery. An **ophthalmic registered nurse** is a registered nurse who has undergone additional training in ophthalmic nursing.

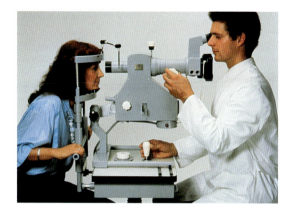

Figure 1.5

An ophthalmic photographer uses special equipment and methods to photograph patients' eye conditions.

Nurses may assist the doctor with other tasks, such as injecting medications or assisting with hospital or office surgery. Nurses and other clinical staff members also may serve as clinic or hospital administrators. An **orthoptist** helps the doctor in the diagnosis and nonsurgical treatment of eye muscle imbalance and related visual problems. Larger private practices and clinics often employ an **ophthalmic photographer**, who uses specialized cameras and photographic methods to document patients' eye conditions in photographs (Figure 1.5).

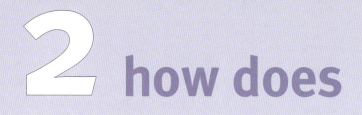

2 how does

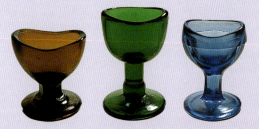

Glass eye baths, ca 1900
*(Courtesy Museum of Vision,
Foundation of the American Academy
of Ophthalmology)*

the eye work?

THE PARTS OF THE EYE

When most people think of the eye, they think of the familiar parts they can see—the colored ring in the center (the **iris**), the black circle in the middle of the iris (the **pupil**), and the white of the eye (the **sclera**). But the eye is much more than just these obvious parts. If you look more closely, you can see a clear, round dome, like a watch crystal, covering the iris and pupil. This is the **cornea** (KOR-nee-uh), which helps focus light rays that enter the eye. Another clear membrane, called the **conjunctiva** (kon-junk-TY-vuh), covers the sclera and the inner eyelids. Normally you can't see this transparent covering. However, it is filled with tiny blood vessels that may swell and show up when the eye becomes irritated, giving the appearance of "blood-shot" eyes. Figure 2.1 illustrates five major parts of the outer eye.

The eye can be described as a hollow ball (the eyeball) filled with fluid. This ball, also referred to as the **globe**, rests in a bony socket in the skull called the **orbit**. Six specialized **extraocular muscles** are attached to each eyeball and the bones of the orbits at various points. These muscles help to rotate the eyes and move them up, down, left, and right.

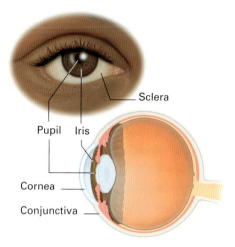

Sclera
Pupil Iris
Cornea
Conjunctiva

Figure 2.1
Front view and side view of the main parts of the outer eye.

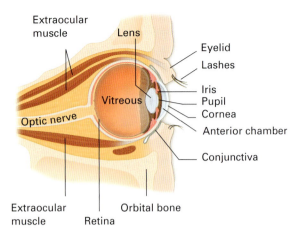

Extraocular muscle

Lens

Eyelid

Lashes

Iris

Pupil

Cornea

Anterior chamber

Conjunctiva

Vitreous

Optic nerve

Extraocular muscle

Retina

Orbital bone

Figure 2.2

The main parts of the outer and inner eye. This side view depicts the eye as it rests in the bony orbit, including some of the extraocular muscles.

The upper and lower **eyelids** are movable folds of skin that cover the outer eyeball. **Lashes** are the tiny hairs on the upper and lower rims of the eyelids. Although not a part of the eyeball itself, lids and lashes are important to eye health. In and around the lids are special glands that produce tears. When we blink, the lids spread tears over the outer eye, keeping it moist and healthy. The lashes help catch dust and dirt that might otherwise get in the eye.

We produce tears fairly constantly while we are awake, so the eye has a system that drains them. This system includes tiny holes at the inner corners of each lid, which are the openings of tubes that lead to the nose. You may recall having to blow your nose after crying, or tasting eyedrops at the back of your throat shortly after using them. The reason is that your tears or the eyedrops have drained through this special system. Together, the special organs around the eye that produce tears and the structures that drain them are called the **lacrimal** (LAK-ri-mul) **system**.

If you were to look inside the eye with a lighted viewing instrument, you would find many other parts, each with an important function. Figure 2.2 is a side view of the eye, with the main outer and inner parts shown. Even the "empty" spaces in the eye are important. For example, between the cornea and the iris is a dome-shaped space called the **anterior chamber**. A special fluid produced by the eye, called **aqueous** (AY-kwee-us) humor, flows through this chamber to help keep an even pressure within the eye. Behind the iris is the **crystalline lens**, which, like the cornea, helps focus light rays on the back of the eye. Behind the lens is another large chamber, filled with a jellylike substance called **vitreous** (VI-tree-us) **fluid**, or just **vitreous**. Vitreous fluid helps the eyeball keep its firm, round shape.

Certain nerve cells in the body are sensitive to heat, cold, or pain. The **retina** (RET-in-uh) is a thin lining on the back of the inner part of the eyeball containing nerve cells that are sensitive only to light. Connected to the retina is the **optic nerve**, which sends light signals from nerve cells in the retina to the specialized portion of the brain that interprets what we see.

HOW DOES THE EYE SEE?

An easy way to understand the process of sight, or vision, is to compare the eye to the workings of a camera. The front of a camera has a clear glass lens to focus (bring together) light rays. In the eye, this light-focusing system consists of two parts: the clear cornea and the crystalline lens. A camera has an aperture, a hole that opens or closes to admit more or less light as needed. The pupil of the eye is actually a hole in the iris that becomes larger or smaller in response to light, acting like the aperture of a camera. The light-sensitive film stretched across the back of the camera can be compared to the light-sensitive retina lining the back of the eye.

Holding a book too close or sitting too close to the television set is harmful to the eyes. Many children with excellent vision like to hold books very near to their eyes or sit close to the television set. Their youthful eyes focus very well up close, so this behavior is natural to them, and it is safe. Children and adults who are nearsighted might need to get close to a book or television set to see clearly. Doing so does not cause or worsen nearsightedness or any other kind of eye problem. An ophthalmologist can test for nearsightedness and can prescribe glasses or contact lenses to correct the problem.

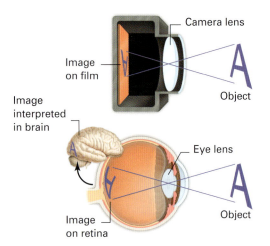

Camera lens

Image on film

Image interpreted in brain

Object

Eye lens

Image on retina

Object

Figure 2.3

The eye operates in much the same way as a camera.

As with a camera, we begin forming a visual image by pointing our eye's focusing system (cornea and lens) toward an object. Light rays reflected off that object are focused first by the cornea, then by the lens. Between the two, the aperture (pupil) controls the amount of light that enters. In the process, the light rays cross behind the lens and are duplicated upside down on the film (in the camera) or the retina (in the eye). While we would then take our camera's film to a processor for developing and printing, the optic nerve and the brain act as the processors of the visual image received by the retina. In giving us the "picture" of what we have seen, the brain turns the visual image right side up again. Figure 2.3 compares how a camera and an eye process light to form a visual image.

WHAT IS VISION?

Most people think of vision as the ability to see objects in front of us. This **central vision** is indeed an important part of sight. It helps us read, sew, paint, or watch a movie. But have you ever noticed an indistinct shadow or movement of something and said, "I saw it out of the corner of my eye"? When this happens, you are experiencing **side vision**, or **peripheral vision**.

To demonstrate the difference, look at the words "central vision" in Figure 2.4 below from a distance of about 1 foot. When you look straight at these words, you can read them clearly, using your central vision. At the same time, you also can see white shapes on either side and perhaps even tell they are words, but you can't actually read them while you are looking at the center of the picture. This is peripheral vision. With it, you can make out shapes and forms but not detail. Still, peripheral vision is important in keeping us aware of our surroundings. As you might expect, we use the central portion of the retina for detailed, central vision and the outer portions of the retina for peripheral vision.

We have a third kind of vision, called **three-dimensional vision**, **stereopsis** (steh-ree-OP-sis), or **depth perception**. With this type of sight, the two eyes view one object, each from a slightly different angle, and the brain then blends these two views to tell us about the dimensions of the object we're looking at—whether it's flat (like a sheet of paper), spherical (like a baseball), or some other shape. This type of vision helps us move around in space and determine our relationship to other three-dimensional objects.

Figure 2.4
Central vision and side, or peripheral, vision are two types of vision we have.

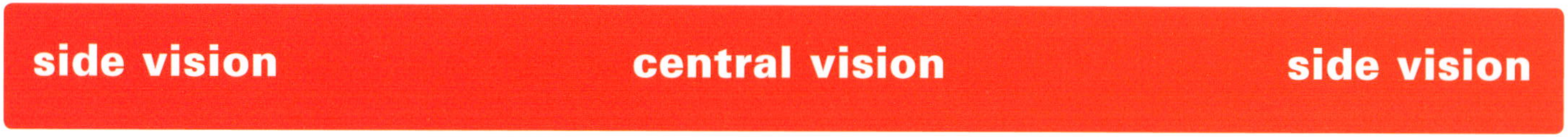

side vision   central vision   side vision

Yet another type of vision exists: **color vision**. Very few people are truly color-blind, meaning they see things only in black and white. Most people with color vision problems simply see things containing the color red or green as less bright than other people see them. A problem with color vision is usually passed on to a person by the mother, and it usually occurs in males. Color vision defects also sometimes occur as a result of disease. Although very little can be done to improve poor color vision, people with a color vision problem usually adjust to it without difficulty.

WHAT IS BLINDNESS?

Many people think that anyone with impaired vision is "blind." But just as there is more than one kind of vision, there is more than one kind of "blindness." Any of these visual impairments may be physical handicaps, but they are not necessarily completely disabling.

Total blindness may be thought of as the absence of vision or the inability to perceive light. Partial blindness may involve having good central vision but poor or no side vision—or the opposite. Some people have permanently cloudy or fuzzy vision because of disease or aging, but they can read or see shapes with the help of special lenses or other devices. Other people lack vision in only one eye as the result of a birth defect, accident, or disease but have excellent vision in the other eye.

The term "legal blindness" is simply a way to define visual ability that is below a certain measurable range or level of sharpness. The concept is useful in helping doctors, social service agencies, and others to provide care for visually impaired people. However, only about 10% of all legally blind persons are totally without sight.

The most important thing to remember about visual impairment is that it is not necessarily totally disabling. A great many people with no sight or partial sight function very well in a variety of day-to-day activities. They all wish to be treated by those they meet with the same thoughtfulness and consideration given to people who have excellent vision. Many will appreciate being warned of your approach by a friendly "hello," so they are not startled. It is also important to remember that people with less-than-perfect sight are usually not deaf, nor are they necessarily less intelligent than people with normal vision. There is no need to shout when speaking with them or to "talk down" to them.

With so many vital components of the eye, and so many aspects to visual ability, it's no wonder that so much effort and so many different kinds of professionals are involved in preserving eyesight and maintaining eye health.

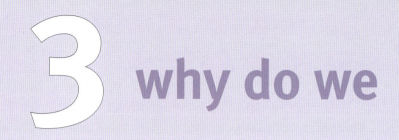

3 why do we

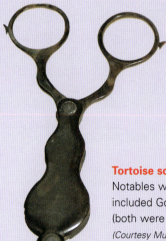

Tortoise scissor glasses, ca 1780 (French)
Notables who used scissor glasses
included Goethe and Napoleon Bonaparte
(both were myopic).
*(Courtesy Museum of Vision,
Foundation of the American Academy
of Ophthalmology)*

need eyeglasses?

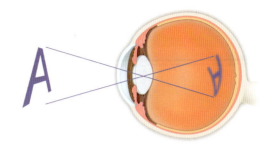

Figure 3.1

In myopia, or nearsightedness, clear images fall in front of the retina, so that distant objects are blurred. The brain "reads" the image right side up.

BASIC REFRACTIVE ERRORS

Millions of people worldwide wear eyeglasses or contact lenses to improve eyesight. Most often, people need glasses or contacts because of some irregularity in the shape of their eyeball or cornea. The problems of blurred eyesight caused by these irregularities are known as **refractive errors**.

Recall that the eye's cornea and lens focus, or bring together, light rays onto the retina to produce a clear image (Figure 2.3 in Chapter 2). If the eyeball is too long for the focusing system, the focused light rays—and the clearest image—will fall *in front of* the retina (Figure 3.1). People with a longer eyeball might not be able to read a street sign from half a block away, but they would have no trouble reading a book held close to their eyes. In other words, they cannot clearly see objects in the distance, but they can see near objects. This type of refractive error is called **myopia** (my-OH-pee-uh), or **nearsightedness**.

The opposite situation also can occur. If the eyeball is too short for the focusing system, light rays focused by the cornea and lens form a clear image that will fall *behind* the retina (Figure 3.2). This condition is known as **hyperopia** (hy-per-OH-peeuh).

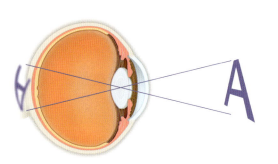

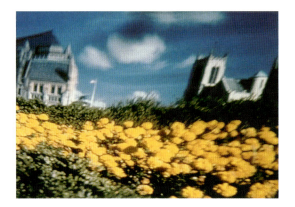

Figure 3.2 (left)
In hyperopia, or farsightedness, clear images fall behind the retina, so that vision is blurred, particularly up close. The brain "reads" the image right side up.

Figure 3.3 (right)
Astigmatism can make both near and distant objects appear blurry and distorted.

Because people with hyperopia see better at a distance than they do up close, the term **farsightedness** is often used to describe the condition. Like nearsighted people, farsighted people also have blurred vision, but most often only when they try to see or read something close up. They usually can see faraway objects clearly.

A third kind of refractive error occurs when the cornea is not perfectly round and smooth. This kind of cornea scatters light rays to different points and prevents the rays from focusing on the retina. The word **astigmatism** (uh-STIG-muh-tizm) is used to describe this condition. It comes from Greek words meaning "no spot of focus." With astigmatism, vision is blurred and objects viewed seem distorted, broader, or longer than they really are (Figure 3.3). Astigmatism can occur alone or in combination with farsightedness or nearsightedness.

As people get older, many parts of the body change and lose their flexibility. The eyes are no exception. In younger people, the eye's lens is flexible. It can easily change its shape to help us focus on objects at different distances. As we age, the lens slowly begins to lose this ability. Starting at about age 40, many people who never needed glasses before find that they now need them to read or do other close work. The name for this kind of refractive error is **presbyopia** (prez-bee-OH-pee-uh). It comes from Greek words meaning "old sight."

VISION TESTING

Anyone who has ever had an eye test at school or at the doctor's office probably remembers being seated at a distance from an **eye chart**, a printed chart of letters, numbers, or symbols in different sizes, and being asked to read as many of the letters or numbers as possible (Figure 3.4). This special examination, called a **visual acuity test**, measures a person's ability to see fine detail with central vision. It tells the examiner how well a person sees in comparison to how well someone with "normal" vision sees.

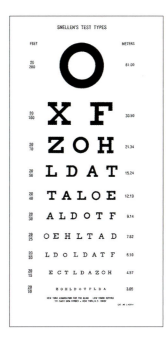

Figure 3.4
A special eye chart is used to test visual acuity.

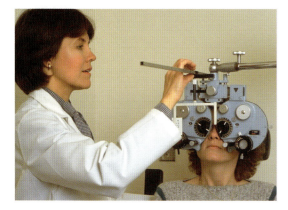

Figure 3.5

In refraction, different lenses are set before the eyes, and the examiner measures the effect.

If a visual acuity test shows that a patient is not seeing as well as he or she should, the ophthalmologist or an assistant may perform other tests to determine why. One of the ways to determine whether the patient is nearsighted or farsighted and whether astigmatism or presbyopia is present is for the examiner to shine the light from a special instrument into each eye and watch the way the eye reacts to the movement of the light. The instrument used in this test is called a **retinoscope** (reh-TIN-uh-skohp), and the procedure is called **retinoscopy** (reh-ti-NAH-skuh-pee). Today, many ophthalmologists rely on an **autorefractor,** a computerized or mechanized instrument that measures and records the presence of a refractive error.

After that, the examiner places different kinds and combinations of eyeglass lenses in front of the eye and may again use the retinoscope to watch how the eye reacts to the movement of the light (Figure 3.5). Once the examiner sees the eyes react in a certain way to the light movement, he or she usually asks the patient to answer some questions about his or her vision and to read the eye chart again with different lenses placed in front of the eyes. When the patient is able to read the chart most clearly, the examiner makes note of the lenses used. Based on this information, the ophthalmologist writes a prescription for new eyeglasses. This process of using a retinoscope or autorefractor and finding the lenses that improve vision is called **refraction** (ree-FRAK-shun).

HOW CAN EYESIGHT BE CORRECTED?

Everyone is familiar with eyeglasses and contact lenses used to improve vision. These devices use specially shaped glass or plastic lenses to help the eye focus light rays properly on the retina. Eyeglass lenses are held in front of the eyes by a frame that sits on the bridge of the nose. Contact lenses are clear discs that rest over the cornea on a cushion of tears. Together, the tears and the contact lenses help the eye focus light rays properly for clear vision.

Some nearsightedness, farsightedness, and astigmatism now can be corrected or reduced by refractive surgery. In **radial keratotomy** (kehr-uh-TOT-uh-mee), or **RK** for short, the ophthalmologist uses a surgeon's knife to make tiny radial cuts around the visual axis (primary line of sight) of the cornea. Newer methods use high-intensity light from excimer (EX-i-mur) lasers instead of surgical knives. Two such methods, **photorefractive keratectomy** (foh-toh-ree-FRAK-tiv kehr-uh-TEK-tuh-mee), or **PRK** for short, and **LASIK** (LAY-sik) reshape the cornea to correct refractive errors. These methods can improve vision for some people to the extent that they may not have to wear glasses or contact lenses for distance vision.

The basic refractive errors described here are usually thought of as irregularities of the eye and not as diseases. However, many people have difficulty seeing clearly or have reduced vision because of eye disease, birth defects, or the effects of aging that is not correctable by ordinary eyeglasses, contact lenses, or refractive surgery.

Wearing eyeglasses that are too strong or have the wrong prescription will damage the eyes. Eyeglasses change the light rays that the eye receives. They do not change any part of the eye itself. Wearing glasses that are too strong or otherwise wrong for the eyes cannot harm an adult's eyes, although it might result in a temporary headache. At worst, the glasses will fail to correct vision and make the wearer uncomfortable because of blurriness, but no damage to any part of the eye will result.

Wearing eyeglasses will weaken the eyes.

Eyeglasses worn to correct nearsightedness, farsightedness, astigmatism, or presbyopia will not weaken the eyes any more than they will permanently "cure" these kinds of vision problems. Glasses are simply external optical aids that provide clear vision to people with blurred vision caused by refractive errors. Exceptions are the kinds of glasses an ophthalmologist may give to children with crossed eyes (strabismus) or lazy eye (amblyopia). These glasses are used temporarily to help straighten the eyes or improve vision. Not wearing such glasses when the ophthalmologist prescribes them may lead to permanently defective vision.

These kinds of problems, referred to as **low vision,** may affect central vision, but they also may reduce side vision or prevent a person from seeing properly in dim light or in light that creates too much contrast or glare.

Low vision problems cannot be completely overcome simply with eyeglasses or contact lenses. However, many special low vision aids exist to help people use as much sight as they have available. These devices include magnifying eyeglasses or hand-held magnifiers to help people do close work. Telescopes, hand-held or built into special eyeglasses, can provide distance vision. Many people with reduced vision rely on large-print books, newspapers, and magazines. Large-print playing cards, clock faces, and telephone dials also are available. Some people with low vision make use of "talking" books (books recorded on audiotape), "talking" clocks, computers, and other machines.

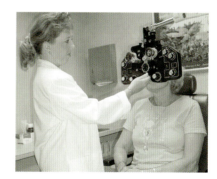

4 what can go

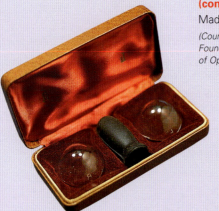

Hard plastic scleral lenses (contact lenses), 1953

Made by Mueller-Welt, Chicago

(Courtesy Museum of Vision, Foundation of the American Academy of Ophthalmology)

wrong with the eye?

DISEASES AND INJURIES OF THE EYE

By now you have an idea of how complex and delicate the eye is. As you might imagine, many diseases and other problems can affect such a complex organ. The exposed parts of our eyes can easily be invaded by germs. The eye may be injured by flying objects or damaged by other kinds of accidents. Disease processes can cause a specific structure in the eye to malfunction. Sometimes diseases in other parts of the body can cause problems in the eye.

PROBLEMS OF THE OUTER EYE

The system that delivers and drains tears can sometimes become blocked. Age or diseases in the body also may prevent a person from making enough tears or making them properly. Without enough tears, eyes become dry and may feel uncomfortably sandy or gritty. Not surprisingly, ophthalmologists call this condition **dry eye**. Usually, artificial tears can be used to keep the eye moist and make the patient feel better.

Another common problem is called "pink eye." The white of the eye becomes very red, and sometimes a clear or milky fluid appears that makes the lids stick together, especially in the mornings. Some people have itchy eyes with this condition. The medical

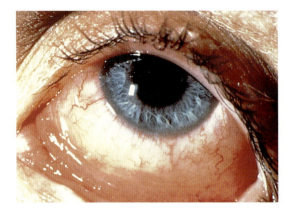

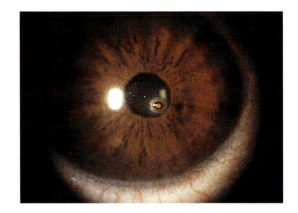

Figure 4.1 (left)
Conjunctivitis can make the eye appear very red.

Figure 4.2 (right)
A small piece of rusty iron has gotten into this cornea. If the iron is not removed, the cornea could become infected.

term for pink eye is **conjunctivitis** (kun-junk-ti-VY-tis), because it is really a swelling of tiny blood vessels in the conjunctiva (Figure 4.1). The swelling might be caused by an *infection* (invasion by microscopic organisms such as bacteria and viruses). Conjunctivitis may also be caused by an *allergy*, which is a sensitivity to something in the environment. The ophthalmologist usually prescribes eyedrops to treat conjunctivitis.

The cornea is the eye's front line of defense against injury and disease. Although the cornea is tough, it still can be easily scratched by a twig, a fingernail, or something as small as a grain of sand. Like the conjunctiva, the cornea can become infected, sometimes because of a scratch or embedded object (Figure 4.2).

Corneal scratches can be painful at first, but they often heal quickly on their own. The ophthalmologist may have to remove the bit of matter that got into the cornea if it doesn't wash out promptly with tears or water. Infections of the cornea can make the eyes very teary, red, and sensitive to light. Once the ophthalmologist has determined what caused the infection, medication can be prescribed to help the cornea heal.

Eyes can become red and feel scratchy just because of smoke, fumes, dust, or eye strain. Many people use nonprescription, over-the-counter eyedrops from the drugstore to clear the redness. These kinds of drops are usually harmless and may clear up redness or make the eye less uncomfortable for a while, but they should not be used excessively. An ophthalmologist should examine any eye that has been red for more than a few days or that is painful or has an unusual discharge.

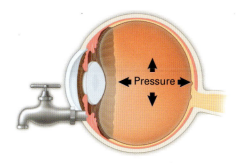

Figure 4.3
In glaucoma, a "drainpipe" in the eye becomes clogged, and pressure builds up in the eyeball.

PROBLEMS OF THE INNER EYE

Glaucoma (glaw-KOH-muh) is one of the most well-known eye problems. It usually occurs when pressure in the eye becomes higher than normal. Pressure in the eye comes from aqueous fluid. This internal eye fluid naturally drains through a meshlike organ inside the front of the eye and is replaced by newly made fluid all the time. If the fluid has trouble draining, eye pressure will rise (Figure 4.3). The high pressure can push against the optic nerve and damage it. When this happens, vision can decrease or can even disappear altogether.

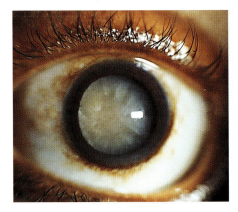

Figure 4.4

A cataract has made the lens behind the normally dark pupil appear milky.

Glaucoma usually is not painful, and from the outside, the eyes look normal. Eye pressure can be higher than normal for years before a person notices any loss of vision. For this reason, ophthalmologists have special methods to measure eye pressure and look at the optic nerve, which they use as part of a routine eye examination. People who have glaucoma nearly always can preserve their vision if the problem is found before it causes permanent damage and if they receive proper treatment. Treatment is usually in the form of eyedrops that help keep a proper balance of pressure in the eye, but occasionally laser or conventional surgery is needed.

Cataract is another well-known eye problem. Cataract is not a growth; it is a gradual clouding of the eye's crystalline lens, which can occur as a natural part of aging (Figure 4.4). If the lens becomes too cloudy, it will not allow light rays to strike the retina properly. To a person with a cataract, objects might appear smeared and hazy, but some cataracts hardly interfere with vision at all. Older people develop cataracts more frequently than younger people, but even infants can have them.

The ophthalmologist can perform an operation to remove part or all of the lens if the cataract seriously affects eyesight. To make up for the visual focusing power that is lost from the removal of the lens, the ophthalmologist usually implants an artificial intraocular lens (IOL) in the eye. Infants and children are usually given eyeglasses or contact lenses instead of an intraocular lens.

The retina is so important to sight that anything that goes wrong with it can seriously affect vision. The disease *diabetes mellitus* (dyuh-BEE-tis MEL-it-us) can affect many parts of the body, including the eye and especially the retina. This eye problem is known as **diabetic retinopathy** (dy-uh-BET-ik reh-tin-OP-uh-thee). People with diabetes may not notice any loss of vision for many years, but the disease can still be causing "silent" retinal damage that may lead to blindness. For this reason, people with diabetes need to visit an ophthalmologist regularly to have their retinas examined.

The retina is made up of several tissue-thin layers. Sometimes an injury or the effects of diabetes or another disease can cause two of these layers to tear and separate from each other. This is called a **retinal detachment** and it can lead quickly to blindness. The ophthalmologist can reattach the torn retina by an operation, sometimes using lasers.

Older people sometimes begin to lose vision when a special portion of the retina becomes unable to function because of age. This special area, called the **macula** (MAK-yoo-luh), gives us sharp central vision. The eye problem is known as **age-related macular degeneration (ARMD).**

Cataracts are removed with laser surgery.

Lasers are high-tech instruments that deliver a beam of special, concentrated light. The light is so intense it can cut or burn body tissue, so it is used in some types of surgery, including eye surgery. Researchers have developed a special laser to be used for cataract removal; however, at present, the procedure has not been widely accepted. Surgical cutting and ultrasound are customarily used. Cataract surgery often involves removing most of a person's crystalline lens. Later, if the remaining part of the lens covering becomes cloudy, a laser might be used to create an opening in the cloudy part to let light through to the retina. This is different from cataract *removal*. This laser surgery is performed only on people who have already had a cataract removed.

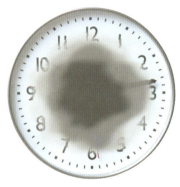

Figure 4.5

Age-related macular degeneration creates
a hazy or dark area in central vision.

Although central vision may be lost, many people with ARMD still have good side vision (Figure 4.5).

Perhaps you have noticed small dark or transparent specks floating in your field of vision. Normally, these **floaters** do not signify a disease or serious eye problem. They are simply particles of natural eye tissue drifting within the eye and casting shadows on the retina. Certain eye conditions, such as a retinal detachment, can cause a sudden and visibly noticeable "shower" of floaters. Anyone who notices such a rapid increase in floaters should see an ophthalmologist immediately.

OTHER EYE PROBLEMS

The word **strabismus** (struh-BIZ-mus) describes a problem in which the eyes are not aligned with each other. One eye may turn inward or outward or in almost any other direction, while the other eye looks straight ahead (Figure 4.6). When the two eyes cannot work together to look at the same object, a person will have double vision—two overlapping or separate pictures of one object. You can get some idea of what double vision might be like by pressing gently on the eyelid of one open eye. The resulting image can be extremely confusing.

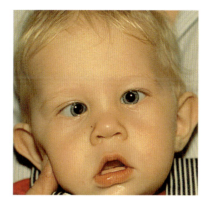

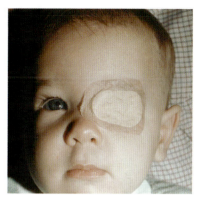

Strabismus in children can create a special kind of poor vision called **amblyopia** (am-blee-OH-pee-uh). Some people know this vision problem better by the common name "lazy eye." Children with lazy eye often have strabismus. Like anyone else, the child finds the double vision caused by strabismus confusing and unpleasant. But unlike an adult's brain, a child's brain can "turn off," or suppress, one of the double images. When a child stops using one eye like this, the unused (lazy) eye may begin to lose its ability to see. The word *amblyopia* describes this type of poor vision. If not treated, the amblyopic eye eventually may become legally blind.

To overcome amblyopia, the ophthalmologist may put a patch over or use blurring eyedrops in the child's better-seeing eye. This forces the child to use the lazy eye, which improves its vision (Figure 4.7). Sometimes eyeglasses also are needed. Children or adults with strabismus may require surgery on their eye muscles, or they may be given special eyeglasses, medication, or eye exercises.

Figure 4.6 (left)
The term *esotropia* describes a strabismic eye that is turned inward.

Figure 4.7 (right)
A child with amblyopia ("lazy eye") may wear an eye patch over the "good" eye to force the other eye to "work."

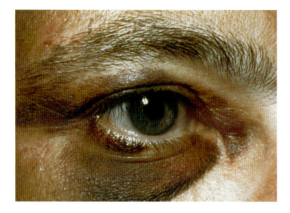

Injuries and many kinds of diseases, especially in the brain, can harm the nerves and muscles that control eye and lid movements. People with these problems may have trouble making the eyes move together properly. They may also have drooping eyelids or be unable to control their eyelid movements. Sometimes a tumor (growth), injury, or disease in the nerves or brain can cause a **visual field defect**, in which a portion of a person's central or peripheral vision disappears. Treatment for eye movement problems and visual field defects ranges from medication to surgery, depending on the cause of the problem.

EYE INJURIES

Not only diseases but also injuries can cause eye problems. Doctors use the word **trauma** (TRAW-muh) to describe injuries such as scratches, cuts, stabs, and blows. Almost any part of the eye can be injured by trauma. Corneal scratches, described earlier in this chapter, are one example of trauma. Another is the familiar "black eye," which occurs when the area around the eye is bumped or hit and becomes bluish black for a few days (Figure 4.8). If hit hard enough, the bones of the eye socket can be broken. A piece of flying rock, wood, or metal might even go deep into the eye. These are all types of eye trauma.

Serious trauma can occur when a harmful chemical accidentally contacts the eye. Many household cleaning fluids, sprays, and powders are strong enough to cause damage if they are splashed, sprayed, or rubbed into the eye. Chemical trauma is a medical emergency. Unless the chemical is removed quickly, the eye may become permanently damaged or even blinded. Anytime chemical trauma occurs, the best action is to hold the eye open to a stream of running water at an eye wash station or under a faucet for at least 15 minutes to wash away the chemical, and then go to an ophthalmologist's office or a hospital emergency center right away (Figure 4.9).

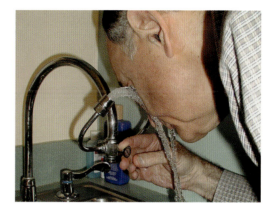

Figure 4.9

Anytime a harsh chemical gets into the eye, the eye should be held open to a stream of running water for 15 minutes, and then the person should go straight to the ophthalmologist or emergency center.

PREVENTING EYE PROBLEMS

Most people visit the ophthalmologist when they notice something wrong with their eyes or vision. However, many serious eye conditions do not cause a noticeable problem right away. Also, the health of the eye can tell a doctor a good deal about a patient's general health. For these reasons, one of the best ways to prevent eye problems is to have regular examinations by an ophthalmologist.

Being careful with our eyes and knowing how they can be harmed can prevent almost all accidental eye injuries. Nearly half of all eye injuries occur around the home. Twigs and rocks can be flung out from lawn mowers. Car batteries can explode if proper precautions are not taken. Explosive fireworks injure many people every year.

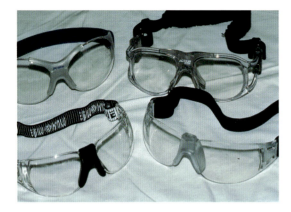

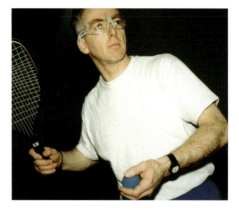

Figure 4.10
Wearing eye goggles can help prevent many
accidental sports eye injuries.

To avoid the most common eye injuries:

• Always keep spray nozzles pointed away from your face.

• Do not put your fingers near your eyes after using cleaning fluids, sprays, or powders. Always wash your hands after using these products.

• Wear protective goggles when working with wood or metal or around anything that can fly or splash into the eye.

• Use safety glasses, goggles, or helmets and face protectors while playing ball sports or other rough sports (Figure 4.10).

• Supervise children at play. Do not let them use darts or other toys that can shoot objects into the eye. Teach them how to handle sharp scissors and pencils to avoid accidents.

The ophthalmologist can treat any eye problem, whether it's a disease or an injury. But safety is the best way to save sight, and prevention is the best treatment for eye injuries.

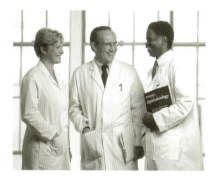

5 the medical

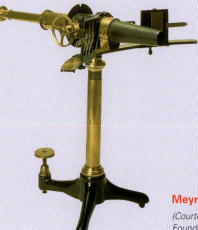

Meyrowitz keratometer, 1880
*(Courtesy Museum of Vision,
Foundation of the American Academy
of Ophthalmology)*

eye examination

WHO PERFORMS THE EYE EXAMINATION?

An earlier chapter in this booklet described the visual acuity examination. Either an ophthalmologist or an optometrist can measure vision in this way and prescribe eyeglasses or contact lenses. But a **comprehensive medical eye examination** is performed only by an ophthalmologist. It includes not only a visual acuity examination but also examinations and tests that can reveal a medical condition threatening to eyesight or general health. A comprehensive examination may reveal a disease or injury that requires eyedrops, other medications, or surgery. An ophthalmologist is qualified as a physician to determine the presence of an eye disease or injury and to prescribe medical treatment and perform surgery.

WHAT ARE THE PARTS OF THE MEDICAL EYE EXAMINATION?

The parts of a comprehensive medical eye examination vary depending on the patient's age, the date of the last eye examination, and other factors. Not every part of the examination may be needed—or performed—during a visit to an ophthalmologist. Some of the specific tests listed here may be performed by an assistant, who reports the results to the doctor.

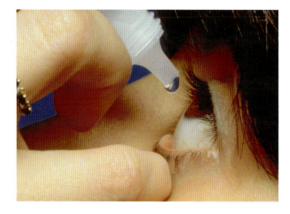

Figure 5.1
Eyedrops are often given during a visual acuity examination to dilate the pupils.

MEDICAL HISTORY Before examining a patient, the doctor or assistant may ask questions about the patient's past and present illnesses and those of the patient's family members. Patients who have come to the doctor because of a specific eye problem will be asked to explain the problem in their own words. Patients also are asked about their current general health, allergies, medications they are taking for any reason, and whether they have had other eye problems or surgery. This medical history gives the doctor a starting point for determining how ill or healthy a patient is. Patients are encouraged to volunteer medical information and to ask questions during this and other parts of their examination.

VISUAL ACUITY TESTING The visual acuity test (described in detail in Chapter 3) determines a patient's ability to see fine detail with central vision. Refraction, the testing process that helps the doctor select the proper eyeglass or contact lenses to correct vision, also is described there. A patient may have a visual acuity problem in one eye but not notice it because the other eye has taken over the work of seeing. The ophthalmologist can determine this problem during comprehensive testing of vision and prescribe correction.

Some patients, especially young people, will be given eyedrops during a visual acuity examination (Figure 5.1). These drops blur reading vision for a few hours. Because the drops dilate (open or widen) the pupils, many patients will find bright light uncomfortable for a while afterward.

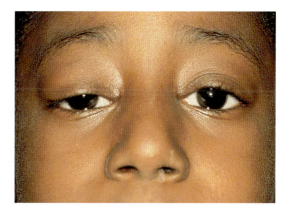

Figure 5.2
A droopy eyelid may have many causes.

EXTERNAL EXAMINATION During this part of the comprehensive medical eye examination, the ophthalmologist carefully inspects the eyelids, the lacrimal system, and the areas around the eyes. Changes in these parts of the external eye can point to diseases not only of the eye but also of various parts of the body, including the brain and certain glands. These changes might include a droopy eyelid (or *ptosis* [TOH-sis]; Figure 5.2), swollen lids, or reddened eyes caused by insufficient tears.

EYE MUSCLE EXAMINATION The eyes can move faster and more precisely than any other part of the body. The ophthalmologist checks that the eye movements are normal by asking the patient to look in various directions. The patient may be asked to cover one or the other eye while doing this. The examination, sometimes called an *ocular motility examination,* helps detect eyes that are misaligned or not working together properly. The doctor also checks the muscles that control the action of the pupils, usually by shining a light into the eyes to see how the pupils react. Pupils that do not react normally can be a sign of eye or nerve disease.

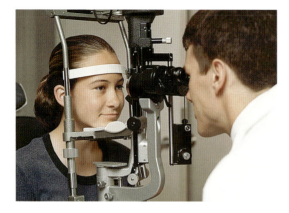

Figure 5.3

The ophthalmologist examines the patient's eye with a slit-lamp biomicroscope.

VISUAL FIELD EXAMINATION The ophthalmologist may wish to test the limits of a patient's field of vision. In the simplest visual field test, the doctor or assistant moves a finger or object from various points outside the field of vision until the patient says it is just visible in the peripheral vision. Other, more complex tests and instruments also may be used. A visual field examination can alert the doctor to the possibility that a patient has glaucoma, neurologic (nerve) disease, or tumors in the brain.

SLIT-LAMP EXAMINATION During this part of the comprehensive eye examination, the ophthalmologist looks closely at the outer and inner eye with a special microscope called a **slit-lamp biomicroscope**, which focuses a narrow (slit) beam of light into the eye (Figure 5.3). Besides the lids and lashes, the cornea, iris, lens, vitreous, and retina can be seen in detail. With a slit lamp, the doctor is able to detect such things as lid infection, inner eye infection or damage, and cataract.

TONOMETRY Eye pressure that is above normal could be a sign of glaucoma, a condition that can lead to loss of vision. **Tonometry**, a test to determine pressure within the eye, is done with an instrument called a **tonometer**. The tonometer tip lightly touches the surface of the cornea and flattens it (Figure 5.4). Another part

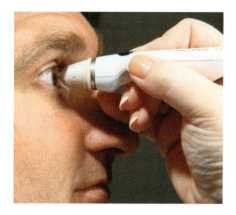

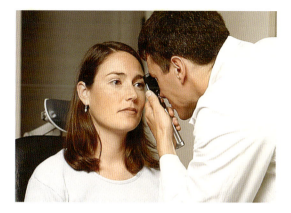

of the instrument then shows a measurement of the eye pressure. Because the cornea is extremely sensitive, patients are given numbing eyedrops for tonometry. The effect of the drops wears off quickly.

OPHTHALMOSCOPY An **ophthalmoscope**, a hand-held *(direct ophthalmoscope)* or a head-held *(indirect ophthalmoscope)* instrument that shines a bright light into the eye, allows the ophthalmologist to examine the retina through the pupil (Figure 5.5). Patients often receive eyedrops to dilate the pupils for this examination, which may blur their vision or make them sensitive to bright light for a few hours afterward. Examining the retina with an ophthalmoscope and interpreting what is seen are among the most important parts of the comprehensive medical eye examination. With ophthalmoscopy, the ophthalmologist can detect retinal problems and other medical conditions such as glaucoma, high blood pressure, or brain tumors and make the proper referral to another medical specialist or prescribe the appropriate treatment.

Figure 5.4 (left)
A tonometer is used to measure pressure within the eye.

Figure 5.5 (right)
An ophthalmoscope is used to view a patient's retina through the pupil.

WHY IS TOTAL EYE CARE IMPORTANT?

As "windows of the body," the eyes can reveal the presence of disease in the brain and other parts of the body. The eyes themselves can become diseased. For these reasons, total eye care is best provided by a periodic comprehensive medical eye examination given by an ophthalmologist, the physician who is legally and professionally qualified to diagnose and treat all eye problems. When a patient has a specific eye problem, the ophthalmologist can perform those parts of the comprehensive eye examination that are needed to determine what is wrong and prescribe the proper medical treatment. To gain a greater understanding of the procedures patients undergo during an examination, new workers in the ophthalmology office might consider asking the ophthalmologist to perform some or all of the comprehensive eye examination on them.

Vision is one of our most important senses. Caring for our eyes is the best way to ensure that we do not lose this precious ability to see.

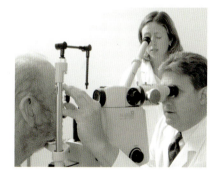

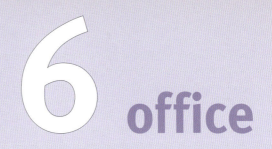

6 office

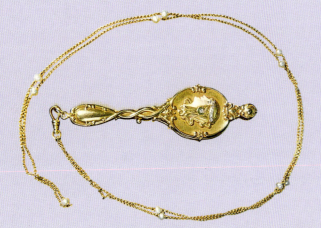

Enamel and diamond gold lorgnette on chain, ca 1910 (American)

Art Nouveau style

(Courtesy Museum of Vision, Foundation of the American Academy of Ophthalmology)

etiquette and ethics

WHAT ARE ETIQUETTE AND ETHICS?

The word *etiquette* refers to acceptable behavior within a society. Often we think of proper etiquette as referring to issues of respect and behavior in public places. *Ethics* is a term used to describe moral behaviors and values. In medicine, ethical behavior is addressed in such issues as full disclosure (informed consent) and honest, clearly defined communication by the physicians and staff—both with each other and with patients.

Because exceptional patient care is the ultimate goal in the ophthalmic office, we must address our ability to treat all of our patients ethically and with the proper etiquette. It is the responsibility of every staff member to ensure that her or his office maintains high standards—from the first contact with the patient on the phone or at the front desk to the technicians, assistants, and physicians working in direct patient care. In this way, patients immediately feel secure and cared for in the best possible environment.

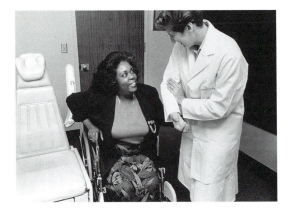

Figure 6.1

A helpful, confident attitude helps patients feel at ease during their office visit.

ETIQUETTE FOR OFFICE STAFF

Medical office etiquette includes attention to issues of courtesy and respect. Most assistants and front office staff are expected to address patients by their proper name, preceded by their title, such as Mrs, Mr, Ms, or Dr, unless the patient specifically requests to be addressed otherwise. Introducing ourselves to our patients by name and professional title is also a common practice. Most offices have guidelines on expected professional standards, but if yours does not, senior staff members can usually provide you with that information.

A helpful, confident attitude when working with patients often helps soothe the fears that many patients have when visiting the ophthalmic office (Figure 6.1). Nonverbal communication, such as facial expression and body language, can express a lot about your attitude and confidence. A smile, positive language, and open body language communicate a comforting manner and often relax nervous patients. Likewise, patients who are fearful about the possibility of losing their sight often communicate negative body language and make us nervous. Understanding this helps the ophthalmic office staff member to respond in an appropriate, comforting manner.

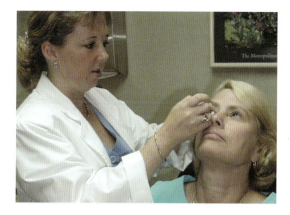

Figure 6.2

Hygiene and neat appearance are important in the office, even for those who don't work this closely with patients.

Etiquette for office staff also extends to the maintenance of a high standard of personal hygiene. Personal cleanliness not only provides a professional environment for patients and coworkers but is also extremely important in the prevention of disease transmission (Figure 6.2). Many eye and systemic diseases are easily transmitted from person to person without proper hygiene and sanitation. Frequent hand washing with antibacterial soap is an extremely effective way to avoid transmission of these diseases. Many offices encourage staff to keep nails well trimmed with little or no polish, limit the use of personal scent such as cologne because some people are very sensitive to it, and keep hair neat and cut short or tied back away from the face so it does not contaminate office surfaces or instrumentation.

Cleanliness and neatness also apply to clothing worn in the medical office. Many offices have a specific dress code, and some require workers to wear a uniform. A senior staff member can help if you have questions about the most appropriate way to dress.

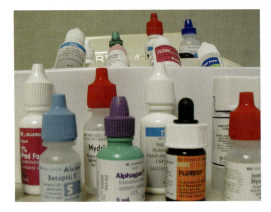

Figure 6.3

Medicines must remain in the office for the doctor alone to give to patients.

ETHICS FOR OFFICE STAFF

Upon graduation from medical school, physicians affirm their commitment to quality ethical patient care by taking the Hippocratic oath. Staff members in a physician's office are expected to uphold this same ethical principle—that is, the interests of the patient should always be the first concern in a medical practice. Ethical care in medicine directly affects the health and well-being of both coworkers and patients. For example, it is critical that medical office workers be honest with their physician employers as well as with coworkers and patients at all times. Mistakes are made, but the detrimental effects of a mistake can be minimized and often corrected if there is immediate disclosure to a senior staff member or physician. The health of patients and coworkers often depends on the honesty and ethical behavior of the medical staff members.

Prescription medications are often powerful and can have different effects depending on the circumstances in which they are taken. This is one of the reasons why the government limits and controls their distribution. Improper use without physician approval and supervision can cause serious harm, or even be fatal (Figure 6.3). For these reasons, it is extremely important that no one, whether patient or staff member, remove medicines of any sort from the office without a prescription or other specific permission from a physician.

Confidentiality is a major concern in medical practices. Having access to charts and medical histories exposes the medical office staff to a great deal of personal information about patients' conditions and lifestyles. It is critical that this information be kept completely confidential; it may not even be discussed with a patient's relatives or friends without specific permission from the patient. In fact, without permission, staff should not even reveal that a particular patient visited the office at all. Personal medical privacy is an individual right and must be upheld at all times. Questions regarding disclosure of medical information to any one other than the patient can be answered by the physician or a senior staff member.

Over time, as you work in an ophthalmology office, you will acquire a great deal of knowledge about eye diseases, treatments, and surgical procedures. Patients often ask medical office staff for opinions on such clinical matters, as well as for opinions on other doctors. It is *always* inappropriate to discuss or comment on other physicians or the medical treatment that has been provided by other physicians. Only a physician is qualified and licensed to diagnose a disease or disorder, and it is illegal for anyone but a physician to practice medicine. Giving medical advice, including commenting on test results, is considered to be the practice of medicine. Although it is sometimes tempting to help a friend or relative, this type of discussion can lead to legal action and can do greater harm to all medical workers. Always refer this type of question to the physician(s) in your office.

Children outgrow crossed eyes (strabismus).

Some very young children have a wide, flat bridge of the nose, which can make their eyes look as though they were crossed. As these children grow older, the bridge of the nose naturally narrows, and eyes that once seemed crossed now appear straight. In these cases, the crossed eyes were merely an illusion, not true strabismus. Children do not outgrow the crossed eyes of true strabismus. In fact, they may eventually lose vision in one eye if the problem is not treated. Parents who think their young child's eyes may be crossed should bring the child to an ophthalmologist and not wait to see if the child outgrows the condition.

Some patients may be reluctant to ask the physician clinical questions directly. In these cases, it may be helpful for you to offer to mention their concern to the doctor for them.

Rules of etiquette and ethics for medical office workers are largely a matter of common courtesy and common sense. If you consider the way you like to be treated as a patient, you will likely make the right choice of behavior. Standards for and examples of etiquette and ethics presented here are general and not necessarily complete. Standards also vary from practice to practice. Consult the ophthalmologist or an experienced senior staff member with specific questions about the policies in your workplace.

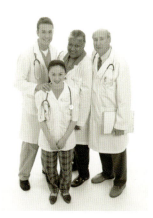

glossary

age-related macular degeneration (ARMD) a retinal condition that causes a hazy or dark area in central vision

allied health personnel clinical workers; in an ophthalmology office, these may include ophthalmic medical assistants, technicians, technologists; ophthalmic registered nurses; orthoptists; and ophthalmic photographers

amblyopia an eye problem in which one eye stops working and, as a result, begins to lose its ability to see; often called "lazy eye"

anterior chamber a dome-shaped space between the cornea and the iris

aqueous humor a special fluid produced inside the eye that flows through the anterior chamber to help keep an even pressure within the eye

astigmatism a refractive error that occurs when the cornea is not round and/or smooth

autorefractor a computerized instrument that measures and records the presence of a refractive error

cataract a condition caused by gradual clouding of the crystalline lens, usually with age

central vision ability to see objects directly in front of the eyes

color vision ability to see color

comprehensive medical eye examination a complete eye examination by an ophthalmologist, including tests of visual acuity and eye health

comprehensive ophthalmologist general ophthalmologist; an ophthalmologist who treats a wide range of eye problems and conditions

conjunctiva a clear membrane covering the sclera and inner eyelids

conjunctivitis a condition caused by allergy or infection; eyes become red and sometimes itchy; also called "pink eye"

cornea the clear tissue at the front of the eye that covers the iris and pupil; helps focus light rays entering the eye

crystalline lens the lens behind the iris that helps focus light rays on the retina

depth perception ability to see objects in three dimensions—height, width, and depth (also *stereopsis, three-dimensional vision*)

diabetic retinopathy a condition caused by diabetes mellitus that affects the retina; may lead to blindness

dry eye a condition caused by insufficient tears due to problems of age or disease

extraocular muscles six specialized muscles attached to each eyeball that move the eyes

eye chart a printed chart of letters, numbers, or symbols used to test visual acuity

eyelids movable folds of skin that cover the outer eyeball

farsightedness hyperopia; a refractive error that allows a person to see distant objects more clearly than those up close

fellowship a period of training following residency during which ophthalmologists learn more about one or two specific aspects or elements of the eye (*see* **subspecialist**)

floaters particles of natural eye tissue in the vitreous fluid that float in the field of vision

general ophthalmologist comprehensive ophthalmologist; an ophthalmologist who treats a wide range of eye problems and conditions

glaucoma a condition caused by higher than normal pressure in the eye; can lead to decreased vision or even blindness

globe the eyeball; a hollow ball filled with fluid resting in the eye socket, or orbit

hyperopia farsightedness; a kind of refractive error that allows a person to see distant objects more clearly than those up close

internship 1 year of hospital training following medical school

iris the colored ring in the center of the eye

lacrimal system a system composed of special organs that produce tears and the structures that drain them

lashes tiny hairs on the upper and lower rims of the eyelids that help prevent dust and dirt from getting into the eyes

LASIK surgical procedure to correct vision through laser reshaping of the cornea; type of refractive surgery

low vision reduced vision that is not fully corrected by medicine, surgery, or eyeglasses and contact lenses; people with low vision often require special aids (such as magnifying devices or loupes) to allow them to function in their daily activities

macula special area in the center of the retina that allows sharp central vision

myopia nearsightedness; a refractive error that allows a person to see near objects more clearly than those at a distance

nearsightedness myopia; a refractive error that allows a person to see near objects more clearly than those at a distance

ophthalmic medical assistant a person who performs a variety of tests on patients and helps the doctor with a patient's medical examination and care in the office

ophthalmic photographer a photographer who uses special cameras and methods to document patients' eye conditions

ophthalmic registered nurse a registered nurse who has undergone additional training in ophthalmic nursing

ophthalmologist a medical doctor (MD) or osteopathic physician (OD) specially trained in the medical and surgical care and treatment of the eyes

ophthalmology branch of medicine dealing with the eyes

ophthalmoscope an instrument that shines a light into the eye, allowing the physician to examine the retina through the pupil

optic nerve the nerve that sends light signals from the retina to the brain

optician an individual trained to design, verify, and fit devices to correct eyesight, usually eyeglasses and contact lenses, based on prescriptions from ophthalmologists and optometrists

optometrist a doctor of optometry, or OD; a non-MD specialist trained to examine the eyes for certain vision problems and to treat some eye conditions; usually prescribes eyeglasses and contact lenses

orbit bony socket in the skull in which the globe, or eyeball, rests

orthoptist a person who helps in the diagnosis and non-surgical treatment of eye muscle imbalance and related visual problems

peripheral vision side vision; ability to see objects to the side when looking straight ahead

photorefractive keratectomy (PRK) surgical procedure to correct vision through laser reshaping of the cornea; type of refractive surgery

presbyopia a refractive error caused by the lens becoming less flexible with age; leads to the need for glasses for close work or reading

pupil the black circle in the middle of the iris

radial keratotomy (RK) surgical procedure to correct vision through radial cuts on the cornea; type of refractive surgery

refraction test to measure an eye's refractive error and to find the appropriate lenses to improve vision

refractive error problem of blurred eyesight caused by irregularly shaped eyeball or cornea; because of the irregularity, light does not focus precisely on the macula

residency 3–5 years of training in a hospital in a medical specialty, such as ophthalmology

retina the thin lining on the back of the inner part of the eyeball; contains nerve cells sensitive to light

retinal detachment a condition caused by separation of the layers of the retina; may lead to blindness if not corrected

retinoscope an instrument used to manually test for and measure refractive errors

retinoscopy a technique to determine the presence and measurement of refractive errors

sclera the white part of the eye

side vision peripheral vision; ability to see objects to the side when looking straight ahead

slit-lamp biomicroscope a special microscope that focuses a narrow beam of light into the eye so the ophthalmologist can examine it in detail

stereopsis ability to see objects in three dimensions (also *three-dimensional vision, depth perception*)

strabismus an eye problem in which the eyes are not aligned with each other, sometimes resulting in double vision; caused when the extraocular muscles of the two eyes do not work together

subspecialist an ophthalmologist who specializes in treating eye problems in a specific part of the visual system following fellowship training in that area of the eye

three-dimensional vision ability to see objects in three dimensions (also *stereopsis, depth perception*)

tonometer an instrument used to determine pressure in the eye

tonometry a test to determine pressure within the eye

trauma injury

visual acuity test a test that measures the ability to see fine detail with central vision

visual field defect an eye problem caused by injury, tumor, or disease in which part of the central or peripheral vision disappears

vitreous fluid a jellylike substance that fills the chamber behind the lens; helps keep the eyeball firm and round

common ophthalmic abbreviations

To save time when writing, most physicians shorten medical words and phrases to common abbreviations. Abbreviations may be used for the names of body parts, diseases, conditions, measurements, and treatments. For example, instead of writing out "extraocular muscles," the ophthalmologist might simply write "EOM." The ophthalmologist also uses special abbreviations to distinguish the right eye from the left eye and to indicate that both eyes are being discussed. Such abbreviations are not only used on patient charts and other medical records, but they also appear on forms used by insurance companies and other medical service providers and on bills or other documents sent by the doctor's office.

Many common abbreviations of medical terms are abbreviations of Latin words and have been in use for hundreds of years. In particular, Latin terms and abbreviations are often used on prescriptions the doctor writes for medications. The abbreviation "Rx," for example, means "prescription" and comes from the Latin word for "recipe." Abbreviations are used to indicate to the pharmacist the number of tablets or capsules or the amount of liquid or ointment he or she should provide. They also indicate how the pharmacist should label the medication so the patient will know how much to take, when, and how often.

Those who work in an ophthalmology office need to be able to recognize the specialized abbreviations used on patient charts, prescriptions, billing forms, and other medical records. This short glossary presents a number of abbreviations commonly encountered in an ophthalmology office.

ABBREVIATIONS USED ON PATIENT CHARTS AND RECORDS

cc *(cum correctio)* with correction; indicates that a vision measurement was made with the patient wearing eyeglasses or contact lenses

CF counts-fingers vision; used to describe a patient who has only enough vision to count the number of fingers the examiner displays

CL contact lens

D diopter; the unit of measure of the power ("strength") of a lens; also indicated by the symbol △

Dx diagnosis

ECCE extracapsular cataract extraction; the surgical removal of a cataract that leaves a portion of the lens intact

EOM extraocular muscles

ET esotropia; eyes turning inward, or crossed eyes

HM hand-movement vision; used to describe a patient who has only enough vision to detect movement of the examiner's hand

Hx history; a patient's medical/ocular history

IOL intraocular lens; an artificial lens surgically implanted to replace the natural lens (usually surgically removed because of cataract)

IOP intraocular pressure

IPD interpupillary distance; the measurement from one pupil to the other; used for prescribing eyeglass lenses; sometimes abbreviated PD

LP light perception; used to describe a patient's ability to see only light

m meter; the basic unit of length in the metric system of measurement; equivalent to 39.37 inches in the English system

mm millimeter; 1/1000 of a meter (m)

NLP no light perception; used to describe a patient who is blind, not able to detect light

OD *(oculus dexter)* right eye

OS *(oculus sinister)* left eye

OU *(oculi uterque)* both eyes, considered together or separately

ABBREVIATIONS USED ON PATIENT CHARTS AND RECORDS *(continued)*

PH pinhole; a measurement used in visual acuity testing

PERRL pupils equal, round, and reactive to light; used to describe the normal appearance and function of pupils

RAPD relative afferent pupillary defect; an abnormal reaction of the pupils to light

sc *(sine correctio)* without correction; indicates that a vision measurement was made with the patient not wearing eyeglasses or contact lenses

Sx symptoms

VA visual acuity

XT exotropia; eyes turning outward, or "wall-eyed"

ABBREVIATIONS USED ON PRESCRIPTIONS FOR MEDICATIONS

ac *(ante cibum)* before meals

bid *(bis in die)* twice a day

g gram; the unit of weight in the metric system of measurement; equivalent to 0.035 ounce in the English system

gtt *(guttae)* drops, of liquid medication

hs *(hora somni)* at bedtime

mg milligram; 1/1000 of a gram (g)

pc *(post cibum)* after meals

prn *(pro re nata)* as needed

qd *(quaque die)* every day

qh *(quaque hora)* every hour

qid *(quater in die)* 4 times a day

qqh *(quaque quarta hora)* every 4 hours; sometimes abbreviated q4h

Rx *(recipe)* prescription for medication

tid *(ter in die)* 3 times a day

ung *(unguentum)* ointment

suggested resources

Beginning ophthalmic assistants and nonclinical office staff may find the materials listed here useful as an overview of some of the many specialized activities that take place in the ophthalmology office.

FROM THE AMERICAN ACADEMY OF OPHTHALMOLOGY

Eye Exam: The Essentials. By Mansoor Movaghar, MD, and Mary Gilbert Lawrence, MD, MPH. 2001, 39-minute videotape. Takes the viewer through the components of an ocular examination of an adult or child, including visual acuity testing, the external examination, pupils, motility testing, and dilated direct ophthalmoscopy.

Fundamentals of Ophthalmic Medical Assisting. By Lindreth DuBois, MEd, MMSc, CO, COMT. 1999, 40-minute videotape. Shows newly trained ophthalmic medical personnel how to perform a variety of basic tests so they can assume greater clinical responsibility.

Ophthalmic Medical Assisting: An Independent Study Course. 3rd ed, revised. 2002, 320-page text. Presents up-to-date principles and practices in ophthalmic medical assisting, including step-by-step instructions for performing basic assistant tasks. Heavily illustrated in color and black-and-white. A separate examination booklet for this text is available. Students study the text and complete the examination on their own, then mail the examination answer sheet to the Academy for scoring. A passing score on the examination partially fulfills the requirements for applying to take the certified ophthalmic assistant examination offered by the Joint Commission on Allied Health Personnel in Ophthalmology.

FROM OTHER SOURCES

Dictionary of Eye Terminology. 4th ed. Edited by Barbara Cassin and Melvin L. Rubin, MD. Gainesville, FL: Triad; 2001. A compact, useful dictionary containing helpful diagrams.

Fundamentals for Ophthalmic Technical Personnel. By Barbara Cassin. Philadelphia: WB Saunders; 1995.

The Ophthalmic Assistant: A Guide for Ophthalmic Medical Personnel. 7th ed. By Harold A. Stein, MD; Bernard J. Slatt, MD; and Raymond M. Stein, MD. St Louis: Mosby; 2000. A broad coverage of the field of ophthalmic medical assisting, heavily illustrated with diagrams and photographs.

In addition, the Joint Commission on Allied Health Personnel in Ophthalmology (JCAHPO), an organization that promotes the education and utilization of certified allied health professionals in ophthalmology offices, and the Association of Technical Personnel in Ophthalmology (ATPO), the national association for ophthalmic medical personnel, are valuable sources of information on professional development and certification of ophthalmic medical assistants, technicians, and technologists. To request information, contact

Joint Commission on Allied Health Personnel
   in Ophthalmology
2025 Woodlane Drive
St Paul, MN 55125-2995
800-284-3937 or 651-731-2944
www.jcahpo.org

Association of Technical Personnel in Ophthalmology
2025 Woodlane Drive
St. Paul, MN 55125
800-482-4858
www.atpo.org